Vegan Cookbook 2021

The Last cookbook guide on how to effectively lose weight fast with Easy and Affordable Recipes for beginners and advanced

Written By

JANE BRACE

Table of Contents

VEGAN CLASSICS

IMPRESSIVE MEALS THAT WILL LEAVE THEM WITH ONLY GOOD THINGS TO SAY ABOUT YOU

IN THIS CHAPTER

Balsamic-Roasted Beet & Cheese Galette

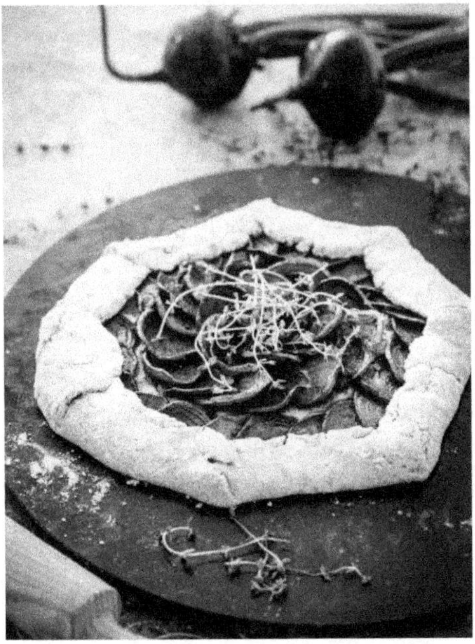

SERVES 4

PREP TIME: 20 minutes (not including time to make Mixed Herb Cheese Sauce)
ACTIVE TIME: 70 minutes
INACTIVE TIME: 40 minutes

crust

¼ cup unsweetened nondairy milk (soy-free if necessary)

3 tablespoons aquafaba

1½ cups unbleached all-purpose flour (or gluten-free flour blend, soy-free if necessary), plus more for the work surface

1 tablespoon coconut sugar

½ teaspoon salt

½ teaspoon baking soda

½ teaspoon xanthan gum (exclude if using all-purpose flour or if your gluten-free blend includes it)

8 tablespoons very cold vegan butter (soy-free if necessary; see Tip)

filling

Olive oil spray

2 medium red beets, peeled and very thinly sliced (see Tip)

2 medium golden beets, peeled and very thinly sliced (see Tip)

6 tablespoons balsamic vinegar

2 tablespoons coconut sugar

Salt and black pepper to taste

Mixed Herb Cheese Sauce, Spread Variation

Fresh thyme leaves

1. To make the crust : In a small cup or bowl, combine the milk and aquafaba. Set aside.

2. In a large bowl, whisk together the flour, coconut sugar, salt, baking soda, and xanthan gum (if using). Using a pastry cutter or fork, cut the butter into the flour until it's evenly incorporated and the mixture resembles small peas. Slowly pour in the milk mixture until the dough just comes together. Turn the dough out onto a floured surface and work it into a roughly 2-inch-thick disk. Wrap the dough in plastic wrap and refrigerate for at least 30 minutes. (This can be done 1 to 3 days in advance.)

3. While the dough is chilling, **make the filling** : Preheat the oven to 400°F . Lightly spray two 9 × 13-inch (23 × 33-cm) baking dishes with olive oil. Spread out the red beet slices in one dish and the golden beets in the other (you can do them all in one, but the red beets will stain the golden beets). Drizzle 3 tablespoons of the vinegar over each set of beets, then add 1 tablespoon coconut sugar per dish and top with salt and pepper. Toss to coat, then spread out the slices again (it's okay if they overlap). Bake for about 15 minutes, flipping once halfway through. The beets will be undercooked, which is okay. Remove them from the oven and set aside.

4. Reduce the temperature to 350°F. Line a baking sheet, pizza pan, or pizza stone with parchment paper or a silicone baking mat.

5. Once the dough has chilled for at least 30 minutes, remove it from the refrigerator. Remove the plastic wrap (set it aside for now) and place the dough on a floured surface. Turn it over so both sides are lightly floured. If the dough is hard, knead it lightly with your hands to make it pliable. If it's too dry and begins to crack, sprinkle with a couple of drops of water. Lay the plastic wrap on top of the dough and use a rolling pin to roll it out until it's a circle about 10 inches in diameter and ¼ inch (6 mm) thick. Gently transfer the dough to the prepared baking sheet, pan, or stone. (I do this by scooting a thin, rimless baking sheet under the dough to transport it to the other baking sheet; a pizza peel may also work.)

6. Spread the cheese on top of the dough, leaving about 1½ inches around the perimeter. Lay the beet slices on top of the cheese. You can lay them out willy-nilly or in a pretty pattern—your choice. If there is any liquid in the baking dish, pour it over the beets. Fold the edges of the dough over the beets.

7. Bake for 35 to 40 minutes, until the dough is golden brown. Remove from the oven, slice, and serve topped with fresh thyme. Leftovers will keep in an airtight container in the fridge for up to 2 days.

TIP

- About 10 minutes before using vegan butter, stick it in the freezer so it gets extra cold.

- When slicing your beets, it's best to use a mandoline to get superthin slices.

French Onion Soup

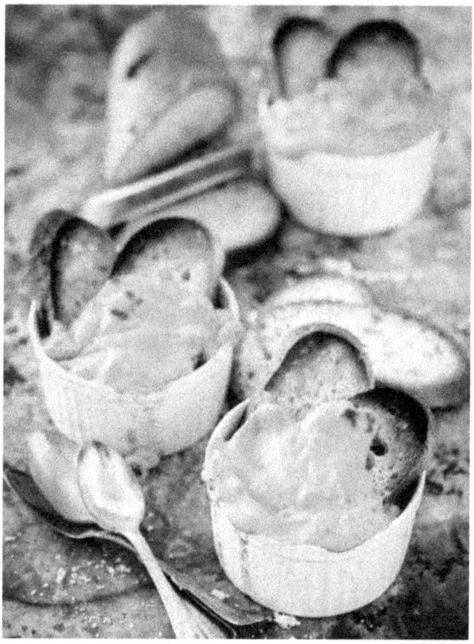

SERVES 6

PREP TIME: 30 minutes (not including time to make Smoky Gouda Cheese Sauce)
ACTIVE TIME: 60 minutes

4 tablespoons vegan butter (soy-free if necessary)

6 medium yellow onions, halved and very thinly sliced

2 garlic cloves, minced

1 tablespoon fresh thyme leaves

2 bay leaves

1 cup vegan dry white wine

2 tablespoons oat flour (certified gluten-free if necessary)

2 quarts low-sodium vegetable broth

1 tablespoon nutritional yeast, optional

Salt and black pepper to taste

1 vegan baguette, sliced (gluten-free if necessary)

Smoked Gouda Cheese Sauce, "Melty" Variation (see Tip)

Chopped fresh parsley, optional

1. Melt the butter in a large pot or Dutch oven over medium heat. Add the onions and cook for 20 to 25 minutes, stirring every so often, until browned and caramelized. Add the garlic, thyme, and bay leaves and cook for 2 to 3 minutes more, until the garlic is fragrant. Add the wine and cook, stirring occasionally, until the liquid has been absorbed. Add the oat flour and cook, stirring constantly, until the flour is no longer visible, about 2 minutes.

2. Add the broth and bring to a boil. Reduce the heat and simmer for about 15 minutes, until thickened. Add the nutritional yeast (if using), salt, and pepper. Remove from the heat and discard the bay leaves.

3. Preheat the oven broiler. Arrange six small ovenproof bowls or ramekins on a baking sheet. Pour the soup into the bowls. Place 1 or 2 baguette slices on top of the soup. Spoon the cheese sauce over the bread. Place the baking sheet with the bowls under the broiler. Broil for 3 to 4 minutes, until the cheese is browned and bubbly. Remove from the heat and sprinkle with parsley (if using). Serve immediately. Leftover soup will keep in an airtight container in the fridge for 2 to 3 days.

TIP

Heating the cheese sauce will take 5 to 7 minutes, so I suggest preparing it while the soup is simmering.

Truffled Mashed Potato–Stuffed Portobellos

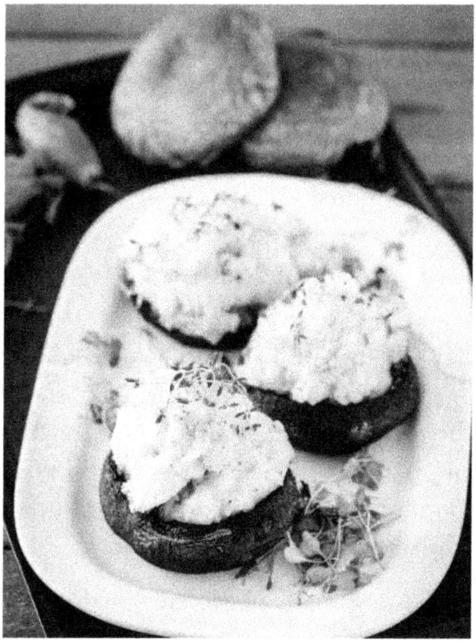

SERVES 4

PREP TIME: 25 minutes (not including time to cook mashed potatoes)
ACTIVE TIME: 30 minutes
INACTIVE TIME: 20 minutes

4 large portobello mushrooms

2 teaspoons vegan butter (soy-free if necessary)

2 shallots, diced

1 garlic clove, minced

2 teaspoons fresh thyme leaves, plus more for garnish

Olive oil spray

Salt and black pepper to taste

½ batch Truffled Mashed Potatoes (see Tip)

1. Preheat the oven to 375°F . Line a baking sheet with parchment paper or a silicone baking mat.

2. Remove the stems from the portobellos and set aside the caps. Dice the stems into ½-inch pieces. Melt the butter in a large frying pan, preferably cast iron, over medium heat. Add the shallots, garlic, mushroom stems, and thyme. Cook for about 5 minutes, stirring occasionally, until the mushrooms are tender. Remove from the heat.

3. Spray the tops of the portobello caps with olive oil and place gill side up on the baking sheet. Sprinkle with salt and pepper, then divide the stem mixture among them. Scoop heaping mounds of mashed potatoes on top. Bake for 20 minutes, or until the mashed potatoes are golden. Serve immediately, garnished with more thyme leaves.

VARIATION

To fancy up this dish, mash the potatoes until they're very smooth and transfer them to a pastry bag. Pipe the mashed potatoes into the mushroom caps as if you were icing a cupcake. Proceed with the instructions from there.

TIP

If you don't already have the mashed potatoes on hand, prepare them while you preheat the oven.

Butternut Squash Risotto with Sage Butter

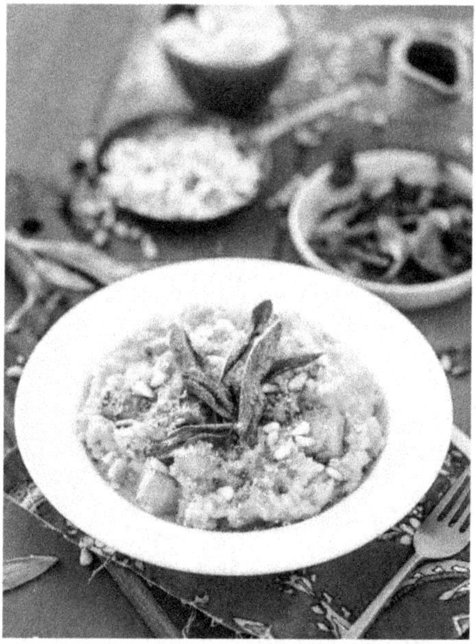

SERVES 6

PREP TIME: 15 minutes (not including time to make Pepita Parmesan)
ACTIVE TIME: 50 minutes

1 butternut squash, peeled, seeded, and chopped into 1-inch cubes

Olive oil spray

2 tablespoons coconut sugar

1 teaspoon ground cinnamon

1 teaspoon ground cumin

Salt and black pepper to taste

6 cups low-sodium vegetable broth

8 tablespoons vegan butter (soy-free if necessary)

1 cup loosely packed fresh sage leaves

4 shallots, diced

1½ cups arborio rice (certified gluten-free if necessary)

½ cup vegan white wine

⅓ cup nutritional yeast

Pepita Parmesan, optional

Toasted pine nuts, optional

1. Preheat the oven to 425°F. Line a baking sheet with parchment paper or a silicone baking mat. Spread out the squash cubes on the sheet and lightly spray with olive oil. Sprinkle with the coconut sugar, cinnamon, cumin, salt, and pepper. Toss to evenly coat, then spread out again on the sheet. Bake for 25 minutes, or until tender and caramelized. When done, remove from the oven and set aside.

2. Once the squash is in the oven, pour the broth into a pot, bring to a boil, then reduce to a low simmer. Line a plate with paper towels.

3. Melt the butter in a large shallow saucepan or Dutch oven over medium heat. Add the sage leaves and cook for 3 to 5 minutes, stirring occasionally, until the leaves are crispy. Use a slotted spoon to transfer the leaves to the plate. Pour half of the butter into a small cup and set aside.

4. Add the shallots to the butter in the pan and sauté until translucent. Add the rice and cook for a couple of minutes, just until the rice begins to become translucent. Add the wine and cook until the wine is absorbed. Add 2 cups of the broth, cover, and cook until the broth is absorbed. Add another 1 cup broth, cover, and cook until the broth is absorbed. Repeat until all the broth has been used and the rice is tender.

5. Add the nutritional yeast, salt, and pepper. Stir in the squash and remove from the heat. Serve topped with a drizzle of the reserved sage butter, the crispy sage leaves, Pepita Parmesan (if using), and toasted pine nuts (if using). Leftovers will keep in an airtight container in the fridge for 3 to 4 days.

Kung Pao Cauliflower

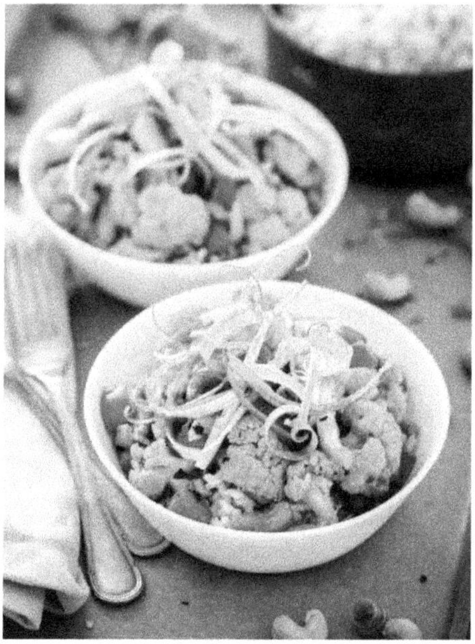

SERVES 4 TO 6

PREP TIME: 20 minutes (not including time to cook noodles or rice)
ACTIVE TIME: 25 minutes

kung pao sauce

¼ cup water

2 tablespoons gluten-free tamari (use coconut aminos to be soy-free)

2 tablespoons brown rice vinegar

1 tablespoon no-salt-added tomato paste

2 teaspoons maple syrup

1 teaspoon sriracha, optional

1 teaspoon grated fresh ginger

2 teaspoons arrowroot powder

1 tablespoon sesame oil

1 tablespoon red pepper flakes

1 cup diced sweet onion

1 large (1½- to 2-pound) head cauliflower, broken into small florets

2 tablespoons liquid aminos (or gluten-free tamari; use coconut aminos to be soy-free)

2 garlic cloves, minced

1 red bell pepper, diced

½ cup cashews

5 green onions (white parts chopped, green parts sliced lengthwise into thin strands)

Salt and black pepper to taste, optional

Cooked noodles (gluten-free if necessary) or rice

1. To make the sauce : Combine the water, tamari, vinegar, tomato paste, maple syrup, sriracha, and ginger in a cup or small bowl. Add the arrowroot and stir until combined. Set aside.

2. Heat the sesame oil in a large shallow saucepan or wok over medium heat. Add the red pepper flakes and stir constantly for about 2 minutes, making sure not to let the flakes burn. Add the onion and sauté until translucent. Add the cauliflower and liquid aminos, cover, and cook for 4 to 5 minutes, until heated through and the sauce is thickened. Add the garlic and bell pepper and cook, stirring occasionally, until the veggies are tender.

3. Add the cashews and the white parts of the green onions, then pour the sauce over the veggies. Cook for 3 to 4 minutes, stirring once or twice, until the sauce is thickened and heated through. Remove from the heat and add salt and pepper, if necessary. Serve over noodles or rice, garnished with the green onion strands. Keep any leftovers in an airtight container in the fridge for up to 4 days.

Creamy Spinach-Artichoke Pasta

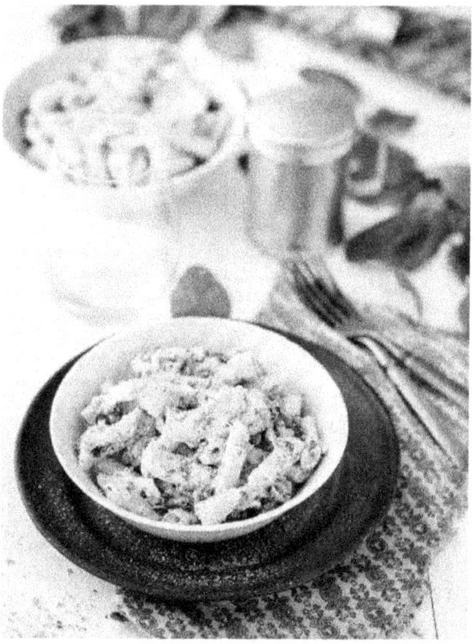

SERVES 4

PREP TIME: 15 minutes (not including time to make Pepita Parmesan)
ACTIVE TIME: 20 minutes

One 12-ounce package frozen chopped spinach, thawed (see Tip)

1 pound penne or rigatoni pasta (gluten-free if necessary)

One 12-ounce vacuum-packed block extra firm silken tofu

1½ cups unsweetened nondairy milk (nut-free if necessary)

⅓ cup nutritional yeast

¼ cup vegan white wine

¼ cup lemon juice

3 tablespoons arrowroot powder

2 teaspoons garlic powder

2 teaspoons onion powder

¼ teaspoon cayenne pepper

1 tablespoon vegan butter

One 14- to 15-ounce can artichoke hearts, rinsed, drained, and quartered if whole

2 garlic cloves, minced

Salt and black pepper to taste

Pepita Parmesan, optional

1. Place the spinach in a clean kitchen towel. Wrap the kitchen towel around the spinach and twist to squeeze out all the extra liquid. Set the spinach aside.

2. Bring a large pot of water to a boil, add a bit of salt, and add the pasta. Cook the pasta according to the package instructions until al dente. Drain and set the pasta aside.

3. While the pasta is cooking, combine the tofu, milk, nutritional yeast, wine, lemon juice, arrowroot, garlic powder, onion powder, and cayenne pepper in a blender and blend until smooth. Set aside.

4. Melt the butter in a large shallow saucepan over medium heat. Add the artichokes and cook, stirring occasionally, for 3 to 4 minutes, until they begin to brown. Add the minced garlic and spinach and cook until heated through. Add the pasta and tofu mixture and stir, cooking until heated through. Add salt and pepper, then remove from the heat. Serve topped with Pepita Parmesan (if using). Leftovers will keep in an airtight container in the fridge for up to 3 days.

TIP

If you can't find a 12-ounce package frozen chopped spinach, 10 ounces will also work, or you can thaw 1 pound and leave a little bit out.

VEGAN SANDWICHES

HEARTY AND SATISFYING MEAT-FREE SANDWICHES

IN THIS CHAPTER

Fillet o' Chickpea Sandwich with Tartar Sauce Slaw

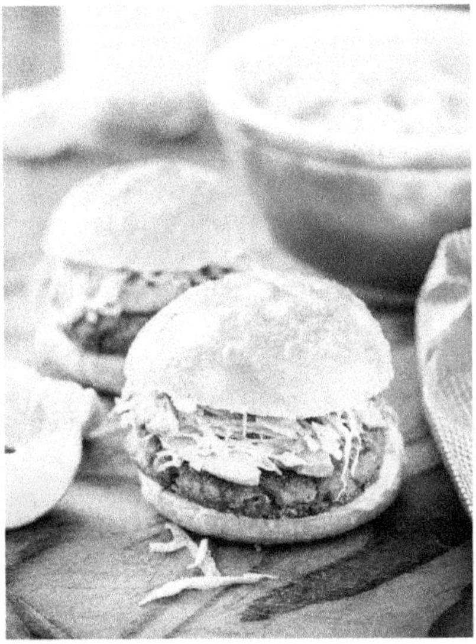

MAKES 6 SANDWICHES

PREP TIME: 25 minutes (not including time to cook brown rice and make Basic Cashew Cheese Sauce)
ACTIVE TIME: 50 minutes
INACTIVE TIME: 2 hours

tartar sauce

½ cup raw cashews, soaked in warm water for 1 hour and drained, water reserved

¼ cup reserved soaking water

¼ cup vegan mayonnaise (soy-free if necessary)

¼ cup lemon juice

1 tablespoon caper brine

1 teaspoon dried dill

slaw

3 cups shredded cabbage

1 cup grated carrot

chickpea fillets

1½ cups cooked chickpeas (or one 15-ounce can, rinsed and drained)

1 tablespoon liquid aminos (use coconut aminos to be soy-free)

One 14- to 15-ounce can artichoke hearts, rinsed and drained

1 cup cooked brown rice

¼ cup + 1 tablespoon chickpea flour, plus more if needed

1 tablespoon Old Bay Seasoning

½ to 1 teaspoon kelp granules

½ teaspoon dried dill

Salt and black pepper to taste

1½ cups vegan bread crumbs (gluten-free if necessary)

Vegetable oil for pan-frying

sandwiches

Basic Cashew Cheese Sauce

6 vegan sandwich rolls or burger buns (gluten-free if necessary), split horizontally

Sliced avocado

1. To make the tartar sauce : Combine the tartar sauce ingredients in a food processor or blender and process until smooth.

2. To make the slaw : Combine the shredded cabbage and carrots in a large bowl and add ½ cup of the tartar sauce. Mix until fully combined and chill for at least 1 hour. Transfer the remaining tartar sauce to a small bowl and refrigerate until needed.

3. To make the chickpea fillets : Heat a large frying pan, preferably cast iron, over medium heat. Add the chickpeas and cook for a couple of minutes. Add the liquid aminos and cook for 5 to 7 minutes, stirring occasionally, until the liquid has been absorbed. Remove from the heat. Use a fork or pastry cutter to gently mash the chickpeas. You only have to mash them a bit; you still want them a little chunky.

4. Place the artichoke hearts in a food processor and pulse 5 to 7 times, until the artichokes are broken down into little pieces but not mushy.

5. Combine the chickpeas, artichokes, rice, and chickpea flour in a large bowl. Use your hands to mash the mixture until it's fully combined and will hold together when you squeeze it. If it doesn't hold together, add more chickpea flour by the tablespoon until it holds. Add the Old Bay, kelp granules to taste, the dill, salt, and pepper and mix until combined.

6. Line a baking sheet with parchment paper or a silicone baking mat. Line a plate with paper towels to drain the cooked fillets.

7. Pour the bread crumbs into a shallow bowl. Divide the chickpea mixture into six equal portions. One at a time, shape each into the fillet shape of your choice (round, square, rectangle), place in the bread crumbs, and gently flip until all sides are covered. Gently shake off the excess crumbs and place on the prepared baking sheet.

8. Heat a large frying pan over medium heat. Add oil until the bottom of the pan is thinly coated. Once the oil begins to shimmer, add 2 or 3 fillets. Cook for 2 to 3 minutes on each side, until both sides are golden. Transfer the fillets to the paper-towel-lined plate to drain the excess oil. Cover with a clean kitchen cloth to keep warm while you repeat with the remaining filets (adding more oil to the pan if necessary).

9. To assemble each sandwich : Spread cheese on the bottom half of a roll and spread tartar sauce on the top half. Place a fillet on top of the cheese sauce, then add some avocado slices, a pile of slaw, and cover with the top half of the roll. Serve immediately. If you plan to eat the sandwich later, store it in an airtight container and refrigerate for up 5 hours. Leftover fillets will keep in an airtight container in the fridge for 3 to 4 days.

The Portobello Philly Reuben

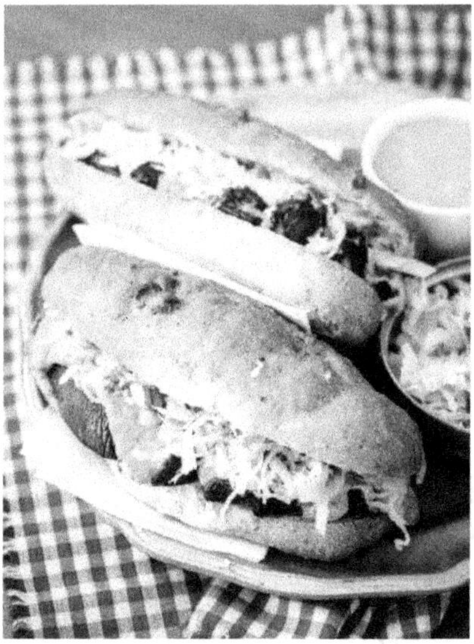

MAKES 4 SANDWICHES

PREP TIME: 15 minutes (not including time to make Smoked Gouda Cheese Sauce)
ACTIVE TIME: 20 minutes INACTIVE TIME: 10 minutes

Russian dressing

⅓ cup vegan mayonnaise (soy-free if necessary)

1 tablespoon ketchup

1 tablespoon no-salt-added tomato paste

2 teaspoons red wine vinegar

1 teaspoon dried dill

½ teaspoon smoked paprika

2 to 3 tablespoons sweet pickle relish

sandwiches

4 portobello mushroom caps

Olive oil spray

2 tablespoons liquid aminos (or gluten-free tamari; use coconut aminos to be soy-free)

2 tablespoons vegan Worcestershire sauce (gluten-free and/or soy-free if necessary)

Black pepper to taste

4 vegan sandwich rolls (gluten-free if necessary), split horizontally

Smoked Gouda Cheese Sauce, Melty Variation

Loads of sauerkraut

1. To make the Russian dressing : Stir together the mayonnaise, ketchup, tomato paste, vinegar, dill, and paprika in a small bowl. Add relish to taste. Chill until ready to use.

2. To make the sandwiches : Preheat the oven to 425°F. Line a baking sheet with parchment paper or a silicone baking mat. Lightly spray the top and bottom of each portobello cap with olive oil and place on the baking sheet gill side up.

3. In a small cup or bowl, mix together the liquid aminos and Worcestershire sauce. Drizzle over the mushrooms, then sprinkle with pepper. Bake for 10 minutes. Remove from the oven and let cool for a few minutes. Slice the mushrooms on a bias into ½-inch strips. Heat the cheese sauce and keep warm.

4. Preheat the broiler. Arrange the rolls on the baking sheet, cut side up. Lay portobello strips on the bottom halves. Spread or drop cheese sauce on top of the mushrooms. Place under the broiler for 1 to 2 minutes, until the cheese is golden and the bread is toasted.

5. Add a pile of sauerkraut onto the cheesy half of each sandwich, then spread Russian dressing on the top half of each roll. Place the top half on top of the sandwich and serve immediately.

BBQ Pulled Jackfruit Sandwich

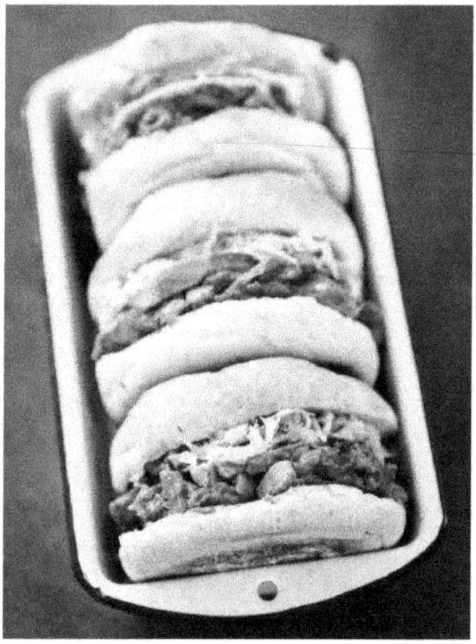

MAKES 4 SANDWICHES

PREP TIME: 10 minutes (not including time to make Creamy, Crunchy Coleslaw)
ACTIVE TIME: 20 minutes
INACTIVE TIME: 20 minutes

BBQ jackfruit

One 20-ounce can jackfruit (packed in brine or water, not syrup)

1 teaspoon olive oil

½ sweet onion, chopped

1 garlic clove, minced

½ teaspoon ground cumin

½ teaspoon smoked paprika

¾ cup vegan barbecue sauce (homemade or store-bought)

1 to 2 tablespoons sriracha

2 teaspoons arrowroot powder

Salt and black pepper to taste

sandwiches

4 vegan sandwich rolls or burger buns (gluten-free if necessary), split horizontally

Creamy, Crunchy Coleslaw

Sliced avocado, optional

1. Preheat the oven to 400°F . Line a baking sheet with parchment paper or a silicone baking mat.

2. Rinse and drain the jackfruit. Use two forks or your fingers to pull it apart into shreds, so that it somewhat resembles pulled meat. It will fall apart even more when you cook it.

3. Heat the oil in a large shallow saucepan over medium heat. Add the onion and garlic and sauté until the onion is translucent. Add the jackfruit, cumin, and paprika and cook, stirring occasionally, for about 5 minutes. Add salt and pepper.

4. In a cup or small bowl, stir together the barbecue sauce, sriracha, and arrowroot powder. Add to the jackfruit. Cook for 1 minute.

5. Spread out the jackfruit on the prepared baking sheet. Bake for 20 minutes, stirring once halfway through, until sauce is thick and sticky.

6. To assemble the sandwich : Open a roll on a plate. Place avocado slices (if using) on the bottom half. Scoop a heap of the jackfruit on top, then top the jackfruit with a pile of coleslaw. Place the other half of the roll on top and serve immediately. Leftover jackfruit will keep in an airtight container in the fridge for 3 to 4 days.

The Avocado Melt

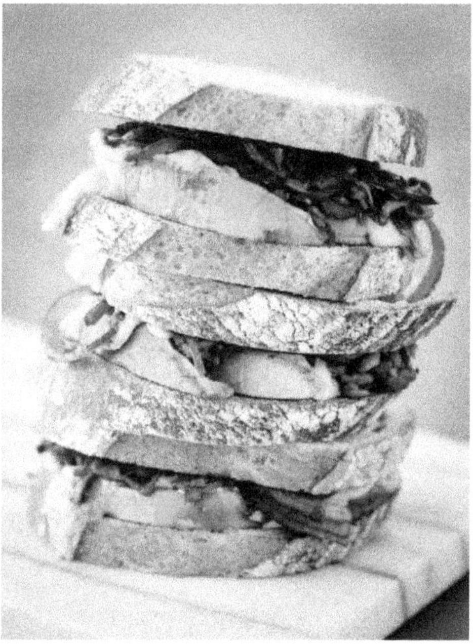

MAKES 2 SANDWICHES

PREP TIME: 15 minutes (not including time to Basic Cashew Cheese Sauce)
ACTIVE TIME: 10 minutes

4 bread slices (gluten-free if necessary)

Vegan butter (soy-free if necessary)

1 avocado, pitted, peeled, and sliced

Salt and black pepper to taste

½ batch Basic Cashew Cheese Sauce, Melty Variation (see Tip)

Optional add-ins: Quick Bacon Crumbles, Pickled Red Cabbage & Onion Relish, sliced tomatoes, chopped green onions

Vegan mayonnaise (soy-free if necessary)

1. Preheat the broiler.

2. Toast the bread in a toaster on a medium setting—you don't want it to get too toasted. Lightly butter the toast. Spread out half of the avocado slices on each of two slices of toast. Place both on a baking sheet. Sprinkle salt and pepper over the avocado. Drizzle or dollop cheese sauce on top. Place the baking sheet under the broiler for about 2 minutes, until the cheese is lightly browned. Remove from the oven and top with your desired add-ins (if using). Spread mayonnaise on the remaining slices of toast and place them on top of the sandwiches. Serve immediately.

TIP

Heat the cheese sauce right before you're ready to put the sandwiches in the oven.

VEGAN BAKING

VEGAN BAKED GOODS THAT YOU DON'T HAVE TO BE A HIPPIE TO LOVE

IN THIS CHAPTER

Peanut Butter Oatmeal Cookies

MAKES 30 COOKIES

PREP TIME: 10 minutes
ACTIVE TIME: 20 minutes
INACTIVE TIME: 10 minutes

1 cup unbleached all-purpose flour (or gluten-free flour blend, soy-free if necessary)

1 cup rolled oats (certified gluten-free if necessary)

1 teaspoon baking soda

1 teaspoon ground cinnamon

½ teaspoon salt

½ teaspoon xanthan gum (exclude if using all-purpose flour or if your gluten-free blend includes it)

¼ teaspoon ground nutmeg

1 cup unsalted, unsweetened natural peanut butter

½ cup maple syrup

⅓ cup unsweetened applesauce (or mashed banana)

¼ cup coconut oil, melted

¼ cup coconut sugar, optional

1 teaspoon vanilla extract

Optional add-ins: ½ cup raisins, chopped peanuts, and/or vegan chocolate chips

1. Preheat the oven to 350°F. Line two baking sheets with parchment paper or silicone baking mats.

2. In a large bowl, whisk together the flour, oats, baking soda, cinnamon, salt, xanthan gum (if using), and nutmeg until fully incorporated.

3. In a medium bowl, combine the peanut butter, maple syrup, applesauce, coconut oil, coconut sugar (if using), and vanilla. Stir until combined.

4. Add the wet ingredients to the dry ingredients and stir until combined. If you're using add-ins, fold them in.

5. Scoop a heaping tablespoon of dough out of the bowl, roll it in your hands to make a perfect ball, and place it on the baking sheet. Repeat with the remaining dough, spacing the balls 1½ inches apart. Use your fingers to gently flatten each ball just a bit.

6. Bake for 10 to 12 minutes, until firm and slightly golden along the bottom. Let the cookies cool on the baking sheets for about 5 minutes before transferring them to a cooling rack. Cool completely before serving. The cookies will keep stored in an airtight container (in the fridge if the weather is warm) for 3 to 4 days.

Salted Vanilla Maple Blondies

MAKES 12 BARS

PREP TIME: 15 minutes
ACTIVE TIME: 15 minutes INACTIVE TIME: 35 minutes

1½ cups oat flour (certified gluten-free if necessary)

¼ cup sweet white rice flour

¼ cup coconut sugar (or brown sugar)

2 tablespoons tapioca powder

½ teaspoon baking soda

½ teaspoon salt

½ cup cashew butter (see Tip)

½ cup maple syrup

½ cup unsweetened applesauce

1 tablespoon coconut oil, melted

1 tablespoon apple cider vinegar

Scrapings from inside 1 vanilla bean (or 1 teaspoon vanilla powder)

1 teaspoon vanilla extract

Flaked sea salt

1. Preheat the oven to 350°F. Line an 8 × 8-inch baking dish with parchment paper. Let some hang over the edges, to make it easy to removed the blondies from the pan.

2. Whisk together the oat flour, rice flour, coconut sugar, tapioca powder, baking soda, and salt in a medium bowl.

3. Use a hand mixer to mix together the cashew butter, maple syrup, applesauce, and coconut oil in a large bowl. Stir in the vinegar, vanilla bean scrapings, and vanilla extract. Gradually stir the dry ingredients into the wet ingredients until well incorporated. Pour the batter into the prepared baking dish and lightly sprinkle sea salt flakes over the top.

4. Bake for 30 to 35 minutes, until the top is golden brown and firm and a toothpick inserted into the center comes out clean. Remove from the oven and let cool completely in the pan.

5. Once cool, use the parchment paper to lift the blondie out of the baking dish. Slice into 12 pieces. You can store the blondies in an airtight container at room temperature, but they'll hold their moisture longer when refrigerated. They'll keep for 3 to 4 days.

VARIATION

▶ I'm sure I don't need to tell all you crazy chocoholics out there that these blondies are just *begging* for chocolate chips. Fold ½ cup vegan chocolate chips into the batter before transferring to the baking dish.

TIP

▶ If you don't have cashew butter, soak 1 cup raw cashews in warm water for 1 hour. Drain and discard the soaking water. Place the cashews in a food processor and process until smooth. You can then add the maple syrup, applesauce, vinegar, vanilla bean scraping, and vanilla extract directly to the processor and process until smooth, rather than dirty up another bowl.

Pumpkin Chai Scones

MAKES 8 SCONES

PREP TIME: 15 minutes
ACTIVE TIME: 30 minutes
INACTIVE TIME: 30 minutes

scones

½ cup unsweetened vanilla nondairy milk (nut-free and/or soy-free if necessary)

1 teaspoon apple cider vinegar

2 cups unbleached all-purpose flour (or gluten-free flour blend, soy-free if necessary)

⅓ cup coconut sugar (or brown sugar)

2 teaspoons baking powder

1 teaspoon baking soda

1 teaspoon ground cinnamon

1 teaspoon ground ginger

½ teaspoon ground cardamom

¼ teaspoon ground cloves

¼ teaspoon ground nutmeg

¼ teaspoon salt

¼ teaspoon xanthan gum (exclude if using all-purpose flour or if your gluten-free blend includes it)

8 tablespoons very cold vegan butter (soy-free if necessary)

½ cup pureed pumpkin (not pumpkin pie filling)

1 teaspoon vanilla extract

Oat flour (certified gluten-free if necessary) for dusting and kneading

icing

½ cup powdered sugar (or xylitol)

1 tablespoon unsweetened vanilla nondairy milk (nut-free and/or soy-free if necessary)

Pinch of ground cinnamon

1. Preheat the oven to 425°F. Line a baking sheet with parchment paper or a silicone baking mat.

2. Combine the milk and vinegar in a medium bowl and set aside.

3. Combine the flour, coconut sugar, baking powder, baking soda, cinnamon, ginger, cardamom, cloves, nutmeg, salt, and xanthan gum (if using) in a large bowl. Whisk together until fully combined. Cut in the butter until all the pieces are smaller than your pinkie fingernail and the mixture has the texture of wet sand.

4. Add the pumpkin and vanilla to the milk mixture and stir until combined. Add the wet ingredients to the dry ingredients and stir until combined. The dough will be wet and sticky.

5. Generously flour your work surface with oat flour. Turn the dough out onto the surface and use your hands to scoop flour onto the ball of dough until all sides are coated. Gently flatten the dough a bit, then fold it over on top of itself. It's okay if it tears, just patch it up the best you can. Flatten the dough again, then sprinkle some more flour on top and

spread it out so that the top is coated. Fold it over on itself again. Repeat flouring and folding about five more times, until the dough is still soft and pliable and doesn't fall apart when folded, but don't overdo it to the point where the dough gets tough.

6. Shape the dough into an 8-inch circle. Slice into eight equal-size triangles. Place them on the prepared baking sheet. Bake for 15 to 20 minutes, until lightly browned and firm. Let the scones cool on the pan for about 10 minutes before transferring them to a cooling rack to cool completely.

7. While the scones are cooling, **make the icing:** Combine all the ingredients in a small bowl and whisk with a fork until smooth.

8. Once the scones are cool, drizzle the icing over the tops. The scones will keep in an airtight container at room temperature for 2 to 3 days.

TIP

For those who are patience deficient, just let the scones cool for 10 minutes, skip the icing, and enjoy right away.

Strawberry-Peach Crisp with Vanilla Whipped Cream

SERVES 8

PREP TIME: 20 minutes (not including time to chill coconut cream)
ACTIVE TIME: 20 minutes
INACTIVE TIME: 30 minutes

filling

Vegan cooking spray (soy-free if necessary)

1 pound strawberries, hulled and quartered

3 medium peaches, pitted and thinly sliced

3 tablespoons coconut sugar (or brown sugar)

2 tablespoons lemon juice

1 tablespoon arrowroot powder

1 teaspoon grated fresh ginger

streusel

¾ cup oat flour (certified gluten-free if necessary)

½ cup corn flour (see Flour Power ; certified gluten-free if necessary)

¼ cup brown rice flour

8 tablespoons cold vegan butter (soy-free if necessary)

½ cup rolled oats (certified gluten-free if necessary)

½ cup coconut sugar (or brown sugar)

½ teaspoon salt

½ teaspoon ground cinnamon

Scrapings from inside 1 vanilla bean, optional

vanilla whipped cream

One 14.5-ounce can unsweetened coconut cream (or full-fat coconut milk)

1 tablespoon powdered sugar (or xylitol)

½ teaspoon vanilla extract

1. The day before you plan to serve, refrigerate the can of coconut cream.

2. Preheat the oven to 400°F . Lightly spray a 10-inch cake pan, pie pan, or cast-iron skillet with cooking spray.

3. To make the filling : Combine the strawberries, peaches, coconut sugar, lemon juice, arrowroot, and ginger in a large bowl and stir until combined. Pour into the prepared baking dish.

4. To make the streusel : Whisk together the oat flour, corn flour, and rice flour. Cut in the butter until no piece is larger than your pinkie fingernail and the mixture has the texture of wet sand. Stir in the oats, sugar, salt, cinnamon, and vanilla bean scrapings (if using), just until evenly mixed. You want it to be clumpy but evenly distributed. Evenly spread the streusel over the fruit. Bake for 30 minutes, or until the topping is crispy and golden. Remove from the oven and let rest for 5 to 10 minutes before serving.

5. While the crisp is cooling, **make the whipped cream** : Carefully spoon the solid coconut cream into a large bowl, leaving the coconut water in the can (which you can totally keep to use for something else). Add the powdered sugar and vanilla to the cream and, using a hand mixer (fitted with a whisk attachment, if possible), mix on high speed until it has the texture of whipped cream. Transfer the bowl to the refrigerator until ready to serve.

6. Serve each helping of crisp topped with a dollop of whipped cream. Both the crisp and the whipped cream will keep in airtight containers in the fridge for 2 to 3 days.

VARIATION

▶ Strawberries and peaches not in season? Try using different pairings of fruit, such as cranberries and persimmons, apples and pears, or blueberries and mango. Just try to replace with similar quantities as much as possible, although if you get a little more or a little less, it's not going to hurt the final product.

VEGAN COMFORT FOOD

HEARTY, SHOW-STOPPING, MADE-OVER CLASSICS TO APPEASE EVEN THE LOUDEST NAYSAYERS

IN THIS CHAPTER

Roasted Carrot & Wild Mushroom Ragout

SERVES 4

PREP TIME: 30 minutes (not including time to make polenta)
ACTIVE TIME: 40 minutes

8 large carrots, peeled and chopped into 1-inch pieces

Olive oil spray

1 teaspoon dried thyme

1 teaspoon dried parsley

Salt and black pepper to taste

3 cups water

2 ounces dried mushrooms (porcini or a mixed variety)

2 tablespoons vegan butter (soy-free if necessary)

½ red onion, chopped

2 garlic cloves, minced

1 tablespoon chopped fresh rosemary

1 tablespoon chopped fresh thyme

8 ounces button mushrooms (or cremini mushrooms), halved

8 ounces wild mushrooms (shiitake, chanterelle, oyster, morel, lobster, etc.; see Tip), sliced

2 tablespoons oat flour (certified gluten-free if necessary)

½ cup vegan red wine

3 tablespoons lemon juice

Cooked polenta or other grain or pasta

Chopped fresh parsley, optional

1. Preheat the oven to 425°F (220°C). Line a baking sheet with parchment paper or a silicone baking mat. Spread out the carrots on the sheet and lightly spray with olive oil. Sprinkle with the dried thyme, dried parsley, and salt and pepper. Toss to coat. Roast for 25 minutes, or until caramelized and tender. Set aside until ready to use.

2. Once the carrots are in the oven, bring the water to a boil in a medium pot, then remove from the heat. Add the dried mushrooms and set aside.

3. Melt the butter in a large shallow saucepan over medium heat. Add the onion and sauté until translucent. Add the garlic, rosemary, and fresh thyme and cook until fragrant, about 2 minutes. Add the button and wild mushrooms. Use a slotted spoon to scoop the rehydrated mushrooms from the water into the pan (do not discard the water). Cook for 8 to 10 minutes, stirring occasionally, until the mushrooms are tender but still hold their shape.

4. Add the oat flour and cook, stirring constantly, until the flour is fully incorporated. Add the wine and cook, stirring frequently, until the liquid has reduced. Add ½ cup of the reserved mushroom soaking water, bring to a boil, then reduce to a simmer. Cook for about 5 minutes, until most of the liquid has been absorbed.

5. Add the carrots, lemon juice, salt, and pepper and remove from the heat. Serve over creamy polenta, garnished with fresh parsley, if desired. Leftovers will keep in an airtight container in the fridge for 2 to 3 days.

Sweet Potato Shepherd's Pie

SERVES 6

PREP TIME: 15 minutes (not including time to make Pepita Parmesan)
ACTIVE TIME: 35 minutes
INACTIVE TIME: 15 minutes

Olive oil spray

topping

2 pounds sweet potatoes or yams, peeled and chopped

2 tablespoons unsweetened nondairy milk (nut-free and/or soy-free if necessary)

2 tablespoons olive oil

1 tablespoon nutritional yeast, optional

½ teaspoon garlic powder

Salt and black pepper to taste

Pepita Parmesan

Chopped fresh rosemary

filling

1 teaspoon olive oil

1 red onion, diced

2 garlic cloves, minced

2 large carrots, peeled and chopped

3 celery stalks, chopped

3 cups cooked great Northern beans (or two 15-ounce cans), rinsed and drained)

8 ounces cremini mushrooms (or button mushrooms), sliced

1 tablespoon chopped fresh rosemary

1 tablespoon chopped fresh thyme

½ cup low-sodium vegetable broth

2 tablespoons liquid aminos (or gluten-free tamari; use coconut aminos to be soy-free)

2 tablespoons no-salt-added tomato paste

¼ cup chopped sun-dried tomatoes (rehydrated in water and drained, if necessary)

¼ cup chopped pitted green olives

1 tablespoon lemon juice

Salt and black pepper to taste

1. Preheat the oven to 400°F . Lightly spray an 8-inch square or 10-inch round baking dish with olive oil. Alternatively, if you have a shallow Dutch oven or large cast-iron skillet, you can use that to cook the filling, then bake the casserole.

2. To make the topping : Place the sweet potatoes in a medium pot and cover with water. Bring to a boil and cook for 8 to 10 minutes, until easily pierced with a fork. Remove from the heat and drain. Add the milk, olive oil, nutritional yeast (if using), and garlic powder and mash until smooth. Alternatively, you can use a hand mixer or food processor. Once smooth, add salt and pepper.

3. While the sweet potatoes are boiling, **make the filling** : Heat the olive oil in a large, shallow saucepan that can go into the oven (or a Dutch oven or cast-iron skillet) over medium heat. Add the onion and garlic and sauté for 2 to 3 minutes, until the onion just becomes translucent. Add the carrots and celery and cook for another 3 minutes. Add the beans, mushrooms, rosemary, and thyme. Cook for about 5 minutes, stirring occasionally.

4. Combine the broth, liquid aminos, and tomato paste in a cup or small bowl and stir until combined. Add to the vegetables with the sun-dried tomatoes and olives and cook for about 5 minutes more. Remove from the heat and add the lemon juice, salt, and pepper.

5. Pour the filling into the prepared pan (or leave it in the Dutch oven). Spread the mashed sweet potato over the top. Sprinkle with the Pepita Parmesan and rosemary. Bake for about 15 minutes, until the top is crispy and golden. Serve immediately. Leftovers will keep in an airtight container in the fridge for up to 4 days.

Lasagna Soup

SERVES 6

PREP TIME: 20 minutes (not including time to make Herbed Macadamia Ricotta)
ACTIVE TIME: 35 minutes

1 teaspoon olive oil

1 yellow onion, diced

3 garlic cloves, minced

1½ cups cooked chickpeas (or one 15-ounce can, rinsed and drained)

8 ounces cremini mushrooms (or button mushrooms), sliced

1 medium zucchini, sliced

1 medium yellow squash, sliced

1 tablespoon dried basil

2 teaspoons dried oregano

1 teaspoon dried parsley

Pinch of cayenne pepper

One 15-ounce can no-salt-added tomato sauce

One 15-ounce can no-salt-added crushed tomatoes

1 quart low-sodium vegetable broth

12 ounces lasagna noodles (gluten-free if necessary), broken in half

3 tablespoons nutritional yeast, optional

1 tablespoon lemon juice

Salt and black pepper to taste

3 cups loosely packed chopped fresh spinach

1 cup loosely packed chopped fresh basil

Herbed Macadamia Ricotta

1. Bring a large pot of water to a boil.

2. Heat the olive oil in another large pot over medium heat. Add the onion and garlic and sauté until the onion is translucent. Add the chickpeas, mushrooms, zucchini, yellow squash, dried basil, oregano, parsley, and cayenne pepper and cook for about 5 minutes, stirring occasionally, until the vegetables are just becoming tender. Add the tomato sauce, tomatoes, and broth. Bring to a boil, then reduce to a simmer and cook for about 10 minutes.

3. While the soup is simmering, cook the lasagna noodles according to the package instructions until al dente. Drain the noodles and add to the soup. Stir in the nutritional yeast (if using), lemon juice, salt, and pepper. Add the spinach and fresh basil and remove from the heat. Serve immediately, topped with a dollop of ricotta. Leftovers will keep in an airtight container in the fridge for 3 to 4 days.

TIP

If you let the soup simmer for too long after adding the noodles, the noodles will absorb more of the liquid and may break apart into smaller pieces. If you have leftovers, you may have to add more liquid when reheating.

Cauliflower Parmigiana

SERVES 4

PREP TIME: 30 minutes (not including time to make Sun-Dried Tomato Marinara Sauce and Basic Cashew Cheese Sauce)
ACTIVE TIME: 20 minutes
INACTIVE TIME: 40 minutes

2 large heads cauliflower (3 to 4 pounds), leaves trimmed

coating

½ cup unsweetened nondairy milk (soy-free if necessary)

3 tablespoons plain coconut yogurt (or soy yogurt; preferably unsweetened)

1 teaspoon onion powder

1 teaspoon garlic powder

½ teaspoon smoked paprika

1 cup vegan panko bread crumbs (gluten-free if necessary)

½ cup oat flour (certified gluten-free if necessary)

¼ cup nutritional yeast

1 teaspoon dried basil

1 teaspoon dried oregano

Salt and black pepper to taste

Olive oil spray

3 cups Sun-Dried Tomato Marinara Sauce (or store-bought vegan marinara sauce of your choice), warmed

Basic Cashew Cheese Sauce

½ cup chopped fresh basil

1. Preheat the oven to 450°F . Line a baking sheet with parchment paper or a silicone baking mat.

2. On a cutting board, hold one cauliflower upright and cut two 1½-inch-thick slices from the center of the head (without removing the core/base of the cauliflower). Repeat with the second head, so that you have four large slices. You can save the remaining cauliflower to use in other recipes, such as the Cream of Mushroom Soup .

3. In a wide, shallow bowl, combine the milk, yogurt, onion powder, garlic powder, and paprika. In a second wide, shallow bowl, combine the bread crumbs, oat flour, nutritional yeast, dried basil, oregano, salt, and pepper.

4. One at a time, place a cauliflower steak in the milk mixture, flipping it to fully coat (use a spoon to drizzle the liquid over the steak to coat it fully, if necessary). Transfer the steak to the bread crumbs, gently flipping until coated. Pat the bread crumbs onto the steak as needed. Place the steak on the prepared baking sheet. Once you've prepared each steak, you can coat the remaining cauliflower slices, if serving.

5. Spray the tops of the steaks liberally with olive oil. Bake for 20 minutes. Remove from the oven, gently flip each steak, and spray with olive oil again. Return to the oven and bake for 20 minutes more, or until golden and crispy.

6. To serve, scoop some marinara sauce onto each plate. Place a steak on top (along with a couple of other smaller pieces, if serving them). Drizzle with cheese sauce and sprinkle with fresh basil.

Brownie Ice Cream Sandwiches

MAKES 8 SANDWICHES

PREP TIME: 15 minutes (not including time to make Vanilla Ice Cream)
ACTIVE TIME: 25 minutes INACTIVE TIME: 2½ hours

1 cup unbleached all-purpose flour (or gluten-free flour blend, soy-free if necessary)

3 tablespoons Dutch-process cocoa powder

1 teaspoon baking powder

½ teaspoon baking soda

½ teaspoon xanthan gum (exclude if using all-purpose flour or if your gluten-free blend includes it)

½ teaspoon salt

1 cup vegan dark chocolate chunks (or chips)

4 tablespoons vegan butter (soy-free if necessary)

½ cup coconut sugar (or brown sugar)

½ cup unsweetened applesauce

2 tablespoons aquafaba

1 teaspoon vanilla extract

Vanilla Ice Cream ; or 1½ pints store-bought vegan vanilla ice cream)

1. Preheat the oven to 350°F. Line two 8 × 8-inch baking dishes with parchment paper. If you have them, use small binder clips to clip the parchment paper to the edges of the dishes. This will keep the paper from sliding when you spread the batter. Set the baking dishes aside.

2. In a medium bowl, whisk together the flour, cocoa, baking powder, baking soda, xanthan gum (if using), and salt.

3. Melt the chocolate with the butter in a double boiler or a heatproof bowl on top of a pot of boiling water, stirring occasionally, until smooth. Remove from the heat. Add the sugar, applesauce, aquafaba, and vanilla. Gradually stir the dry ingredients into the wet ingredients.

4. Divide the batter between the two baking dishes and spread until smooth and even. The batter may be difficult to spread, so if you need to, you can place a sheet of plastic wrap over the batter and use your hand to push or spread it. Bake for 25 to 30 minutes, until set and the edges are pulling away from the pan slightly. Remove from the oven and let cool for 1 to 2 hours.

5. Remove the ice cream from the freezer to soften for about 15 minutes before you plan to use it. Spread ice cream on top of the brownie layer in one pan. Create an even layer that's ½ to 1 inch thick. (To spread it more easily, place a sheet of plastic wrap over the ice cream and use your fingers to pat it down.)

6. Use the parchment paper to carefully lift the other brownie layer from the second dish and place it on top of the ice cream. Gently press down to compress the sandwiches. Cover the pan and freeze for 30 to 60 minutes, until the ice cream is solid again.

7. Remove the pan from the freezer. Use the parchment paper to lift the big sandwich from the pan and place it on a flat surface, such as a cutting board. Use a knife, cookie cutter, or biscuit cutter to cut out your desired sandwich shapes. If using a cookie or biscuit cutter, you will have to gently push from the bottom, underneath the parchment paper, to get the sandwiches to pop up. Place the sandwiches in an airtight container. Freeze until ready to serve, or for up to 1 month.

VEGAN FOR PICKY EATERS

ADAPTABLE MEALS THAT EVEN THE PICKIEST EATERS CAN ENJOY WITH THE REST OF YOU

IN THIS CHAPTER

BLT Summer Rolls with Avocado

MAKES 8 ROLLS

PREP TIME: 15 minutes (not including time to make Quick Bacon Crumbles and Avocado Ranch Dressing or Lemon Dill Aïoli)
ACTIVE TIME: 25 minutes

Quick Bacon Crumbles (or 10 oz vegan bacon of your choice)

1 small head romaine lettuce, separated into leaves, each leaf chopped in half widthwise

2 to 3 Roma tomatoes, seeded and thinly sliced lengthwise

1 avocado, pitted, peeled, and sliced, optional

Eight 8-inch sheets rice paper (see Tip)

Avocado Ranch Dressing or Lemon Dill Aïoli

1. Fill a large bowl with warm water. Make sure you have a clean surface to prepare the rolls on.

2. Dip a sheet of rice paper into the water, making sure to get it completely wet but removing it quickly before it gets too soft. Lay the paper on the clean surface, then lay a few pieces of lettuce on the center of the paper, going from side to side and leaving about an inch of space around the perimeter. Add a few slices of tomato, a few slices of avocado (if using), and a few spoonfuls of the bacon crumbles (or 2 or 3 slices if you're using a sliced variety).

3. Fold the left and right sides of the paper over the filling. Take the edge of the paper closest to you and fold it completely over the filling while using your fingers to tuck the filling in. Continue rolling until the roll is sealed. Repeat with the remaining ingredients. Serve immediately with the Avocado Ranch Dressing or Lemon Dill Aïoli. These rolls are best enjoyed right after they're made but will keep in an airtight container in the fridge for 5 or 6 hours.

VARIATIONS

- For those who aren't fond of avocado, you can leave it out, and switch out the Avocado Ranch Dressing with a regular vegan ranch dressing, or use the Lemon Dill Aïoli.

- If your family isn't into summer rolls, just pile all the ingredients between two slices of bread for a sandwich. You won't get any complaints.

TIP

- Rice paper sheets that are 6 inches in diameter will be too small.

Perfect Roasted Potatoes

SERVES 4 TO 6

PREP TIME: 10 minutes
ACTIVE TIME: 10 minutes
INACTIVE TIME: 40 minutes

Olive oil spray or vegan cooking spray (soy-free if necessary)

2 pounds Yukon gold potatoes, peeled and chopped into 1-inch cubes

4 tablespoons vegan butter (soy-free if necessary), melted (or ¼ cup olive oil)

2 teaspoons garlic powder

2 teaspoons dried thyme or rosemary

Salt and black pepper to taste

1. Preheat the oven to 400°F . Lightly spray two baking sheets with olive oil.

2. Place the potatoes in a medium pot and cover them with water. Bring to a boil and cook for 5 to 6 minutes, until tender. Drain.

3. Spread out the potatoes on the baking sheets. Use a spatula to gently smash each one just a little bit. Pour the butter over the potatoes. Sprinkle the garlic powder, thyme, salt, and pepper on top. Toss to coat, then spread them out again, making sure that the pieces aren't touching. Bake for 40 minutes, flipping them halfway through. Serve immediately. Leftovers will keep in an airtight container in the fridge for 2 to 3 days.

VARIATION

- Feel free to try other seasonings if garlic powder, thyme, or rosemary don't float your boat.

Cauliflower Alfredo Baked Ziti

SERVES 6 TO 8

PREP TIME: 10 minutes (not including time to make Pepita Parmesan)
ACTIVE TIME: 30 minutes
INACTIVE TIME: 50 minutes

Olive oil spray or vegan cooking spray (soy-free if necessary)

1 large (1½- to 2-pound) head cauliflower, broken into florets

3 cups low-sodium vegetable broth

1 pound ziti or penne pasta (gluten-free if necessary)

1 cup raw cashews, soaked in warm water for at least 30 minutes and drained, water discarded

2 cups unsweetened nondairy milk (soy-free if necessary)

¼ cup nutritional yeast

¼ cup vegan white wine

3 tablespoons olive oil

3 tablespoons lemon juice

2 teaspoons white soy miso (or chickpea miso)

2 teaspoons onion powder

2 teaspoons garlic powder

¼ teaspoon ground nutmeg

Salt and black pepper to taste

Pepita Parmesan

1. Preheat the oven to 350°F. Lightly spray a 9 × 13-inch baking dish with olive oil. Bring a large pot of water to a boil.

2. Combine the cauliflower and broth in a medium pot, cover, and bring to a boil. Reduce to a simmer, cover again, and simmer for 10 minutes, or until the cauliflower is soft. Remove from the heat.

3. Cook the pasta according to the package instructions until al dente. Drain. Set aside in a large bowl.

4. While the pasta is cooking, use a slotted spoon to scoop the cauliflower into a blender. (You can save the broth for another use.) Add the cashews, milk, nutritional yeast, wine, oil, lemon juice, miso, onion powder, garlic powder, nutmeg, salt, and pepper. Blend until smooth.

5. Add the sauce to the pasta. Stir until combined, then pour into the prepared baking dish. Sprinkle the Pepita Parmesan over the top and bake for 20 minutes. Serve immediately. Leftovers will keep in an airtight container in the fridge for up to 4 days.

VARIATION

To add some flavor or texture, try adding sautéed mushrooms, caramelized onions, steamed broccoli, or cooked greens.

Creamy Roasted Garlic–Tomato Soup with Grilled Cheese Croutons

SERVES 4

PREP TIME: 20 minutes (not including time to make Basic Cashew Cheese Sauce)
ACTIVE TIME: 45 minutes
INACTIVE TIME: 40 minutes

soup

3 to 4 pounds Roma tomatoes, halved lengthwise

1 teaspoon olive oil, plus more for roasting

Salt and black pepper to taste

1 small garlic head (see Variation)

1 sweet onion, diced

One 6-ounce can no-salt-added tomato paste

2 tablespoons coconut sugar (or brown sugar)

2 tablespoons white wine vinegar

2 teaspoons dried basil

1 teaspoon dried oregano

3 cups low-sodium vegetable broth

½ cup unsweetened nondairy milk (soy-free if necessary)

1 tablespoon nutritional yeast, optional

2 to 3 tablespoons chopped fresh basil, optional

croutons

4 vegan sandwich bread slices (gluten-free if necessary)

Basic Cashew Cheese Sauce, Melty Variation

Vegan butter (soy-free if necessary)

1. Preheat the oven to 400°F . Line one or two baking sheets with parchment paper or silicone baking mats. Spread out the tomato halves on the baking sheet(s), cut side up. Drizzle with olive oil and sprinkle with salt and pepper.

2. Trim the top off the head of garlic so that all the cloves are exposed. Place the head on a sheet of aluminum foil, drizzle with olive oil, and sprinkle with salt and pepper. Wrap the foil around the head so that it's completely enclosed. Roast the garlic and the tomatoes for about 40 minutes, until the garlic is soft and the tomatoes slightly charred. Remove from the oven. Unwrap the garlic so it can cool. Set the tomatoes aside.

3. While the garlic is cooling, heat 1 teaspoon olive oil in a large pot over medium heat. Add the onion and sauté until translucent. Transfer to a blender.

4. Once the garlic is cool to the touch, squeeze each clove over a small plate or bowl so that the garlic pops out. Transfer all the garlic to the blender along with the onions, roasted tomatoes, tomato paste, sugar, vinegar, dried basil, and oregano. Blend until smooth.

5. Combine the tomato mixture and broth in the large pot and bring to a boil. Reduce to a simmer and cook for about 15 minutes, stirring occasionally, until heated through and slightly thickened. Stir in the milk and nutritional yeast (if using) and cook for another 5 minutes. Reduce the heat to low and cover to keep the soup warm.

6. While the soup is simmering, **make the croutons** : Lay out 2 slices of bread, spread them with cheese, and top each with another slice of bread. Spread butter on the outsides of each sandwich. Heat a frying pan, preferably cast iron, over medium heat. Place both sandwiches in the pan and cook for 2 to 3 minutes per side, until each side is crispy and golden. Remove from the heat and cut each sandwich into six squares.

7. Spoon the soup into bowls and top each serving with a sprinkle of fresh basil (if using) and 3 or 4 grilled cheese croutons (or serve them on the side and add them as you eat). Serve immediately. Leftover soup will keep in an airtight container in the fridge for 3 to 4 days.

VARIATION

- If your family doesn't care for garlic, you can totally leave it out altogether.

GAME DAY VEGAN

DECADENT SNACKAGE THAT NOBODY WILL GUESS IS VEGAN

IN THIS CHAPTER

Jalapeño Popper Bites

MAKES 16 TO 18 POPPERS

PREP TIME: 15 minutes (not including time to cook quinoa)
ACTIVE TIME: 25 minutes

2 cups cooked quinoa

1 cup corn flour (certified gluten-free if necessary), plus more if needed

3 or 4 small jalapeños, seeded and chopped

2 tablespoons unsweetened nondairy milk (nut-free and/or soy-free if necessary; see Variations)

2 tablespoons lime juice

2 tablespoons vegan cream cheese or mayonnaise (soy-free if necessary)

3 tablespoons nutritional yeast

1 teaspoon ground cumin

½ teaspoon ground coriander

½ teaspoon smoked paprika

Salt and black pepper to taste

Sunflower or canola oil for frying

Salsa

1. Combine the quinoa, corn flour, jalapeños, milk, lime juice, cream cheese or mayonnaise, nutritional yeast, cumin, coriander, and paprika in a large bowl and mix until fully combined. It should be moist and hold together when squeezed, but not wet like batter. If it's too wet, add corn flour by the tablespoon until you have the right consistency. Add salt and pepper.

2. Line a baking sheet with parchment paper or a silicone baking mat. Scoop about 2 tablespoons of the mixture into your hand and shape it into a ball. Place on the prepared baking sheet. Repeat with the remaining mixture.

3. Heat a large frying pan, preferably cast iron, over medium heat. Pour in enough oil to coat the bottom and heat for 2 to 3 minutes. It is important to give the oil enough time to heat. (The bites will fall apart if the oil is not hot enough.) Check to make sure it's hot enough by adding a pinch of the dough to the pan. If it sputters and sizzles, the oil is ready. Line a plate with paper towels.

4. Carefully place 5 or 6 bites in the pan and cook for 3 to 4 minutes, until golden and firm, flipping them every 30 seconds or so to cook on all sides. Use a slotted spoon to transfer them to the plate, placing more paper towels on top to absorb the excess oil. Repeat with the remaining bites, adding more oil to the pan as needed (allow the oil to heat each time you add more). Serve warm, with salsa for dipping. These are best eaten the same day but will keep in an airtight container in the fridge for 1 to 2 days.

VARIATIONS

- Make these poppers extra hot by replacing half or all of the milk with hot sauce.

- To bake the poppers instead of frying them, preheat the oven to 375°F (190°C), place the poppers on a baking sheet lined with parchment paper or a silicone baking mat, and bake for 30 minutes, flipping once halfway through.

Cheesy Spiced Popcorn

SERVES 4 TO 6

PREP TIME: 5 minutes
ACTIVE TIME: 10 minutes

3 tablespoons nutritional yeast

2 teaspoons chili powder

½ teaspoon garlic powder

A few pinches of cayenne pepper

2 tablespoons sunflower oil (or canola oil)

½ cup popcorn kernels

1 tablespoon vegan butter (soy-free if necessary, or coconut oil), melted

Salt to taste

1. In a small cup or bowl, mix together the nutritional yeast, chili powder, garlic powder, and cayenne pepper. Set aside.

2. Combine the oil and 3 popcorn kernels in a large pot and heat over medium-high heat. Once the kernels pop, add the remaining kernels, cover the pot, shake it a couple of times, and return to the heat. Once the popping begins, continue to shake it every 3 to 5 seconds until the popping stops. Remove from the heat and uncover.

3. Pour the melted butter over the popcorn, cover the pot again, and shake to coat. Uncover the pot and add the nutritional yeast mix, cover again, and shake to coat. Uncover the pot and add salt. Serve immediately.

Chickpea-Avocado Taquitos

MAKES 8 TAQUITOS

PREP TIME: 5 minutes
ACTIVE TIME: 25 minutes   INACTIVE TIME: 20 minutes

1½ cups cooked chickpeas (or one 15-ounce can, rinsed and drained)

2 tablespoons liquid aminos (or gluten-free tamari; use coconut aminos to be soy-free)

1 avocado, pitted

2½ tablespoons lime juice

2 green onions, chopped (green and white parts)

1½ tablespoons plain vegan yogurt (or mayonnaise; soy-free if necessary), optional, to add creaminess

½ teaspoon ancho chile powder

½ teaspoon garlic powder

Salt and black pepper to taste

8 corn tortillas (see Tip)

Olive oil spray

Salsa or dip of your choice

1. Preheat the oven to 350°F. Line a baking sheet with parchment paper or a silicone baking mat.

2. Heat a large frying pan, preferably cast iron, over medium heat. Add the chickpeas and liquid aminos and cook, stirring occasionally, until all the liquid has been absorbed. Remove from the heat and let cool for 2 to 3 minutes. Use a potato masher or pastry cutter to mash the chickpeas into small pieces.

3. Scoop the avocado flesh into a large bowl and mash until smooth but slightly chunky. Add the chickpeas, lime juice, green onions, yogurt (if using), ancho chile powder, garlic powder, salt, and pepper. Stir until combined.

4. Heat a frying pan over medium heat and heat the tortillas, one at a time, for 30 seconds on each side, until soft and pliable. Stack them on a plate and cover with aluminum foil while you cook the rest.

5. Lay out 1 tortilla and spread about 3 tablespoons of the avocado mixture down the center. Roll into a tube and place it seam side down on the prepared baking sheet. Repeat with the remaining tortillas and filling.

6. Spray the taquitos with olive oil and bake for 10 minutes. Flip the taquitos, spray them with olive oil again, and bake for another 10 minutes, or until crispy. Serve immediately with your choice of dip or salsa.

VARIATIONS

- You can make taquitos with a plethora of different fillings. Try Jackfruit Carnitas, 15-Minute Refried Beans with Pepperjack Cheese Sauce, Tempeh Sloppy Joes, or even Scrambled Tofu.

TIP

- Thin corn tortillas work best for these taquitos. Steer away from ones that say "handmade," as those are generally thicker and more likely to crack when you roll them up.

Cilantro Chile Almond Dip

MAKES 1¾ CUPS

PREP TIME: 10 minutes
ACTIVE TIME: 10 minutes
INACTIVE TIME: 2 hours

1 cup raw almonds, soaked in warm water for at least 1 hour and drained, water reserved

1 cup reserved soaking water

1 cup roughly chopped fresh cilantro

¼ cup canned diced green chiles

¼ cup lime juice

2 tablespoons liquid aminos (or gluten-free tamari; use coconut aminos to be soy-free)

2 tablespoons chopped yellow onion

4 teaspoons nutritional yeast

2 teaspoons chopped garlic

1 teaspoon ground cumin

A few pinches of cayenne pepper

Salt and black pepper to taste

Combine all of the ingredients in a high-speed blender or food processor and blend until smooth and creamy. Transfer to an airtight container and refrigerate for 1 hour prior to serving. The dip should thicken as it chills. It will keep in an airtight container in the fridge for 2 to 3 days.

GET-TOGETHER VEGAN MEALS

SPECIAL MEALS FOR FANCIER GET-TOGETHERS

IN THIS CHAPTER

Chickpea Caesar Pasta Salad

SERVES 6 TO 8

PREP TIME: 10 minutes (not including time to make Pepita Parmesan)
ACTIVE TIME: 30 minutes **INACTIVE TIME: 2 hours**

caesar dressing

¼ cup raw cashews, soaked in warm water for 1 hour and drained, water reserved

6 tablespoons reserved soaking water

¼ cup hemp seeds

3 tablespoons lemon juice

2 tablespoons olive oil

1 tablespoon vegan mayonnaise (soy-free if necessary), optional

1 tablespoon nutritional yeast

2 teaspoons vegan Worcestershire sauce (gluten-free and/or soy-free if necessary)

2 teaspoons Dijon mustard (gluten-free if necessary)

2 teaspoons drained capers

1 garlic clove

Salt and black pepper to taste

salad

12 ounces pasta shape of your choice (gluten-free if necessary)

3 cups cooked chickpeas (or two 15-ounce cans, rinsed and drained)

¼ cup liquid aminos (use coconut aminos to be soy-free)

2 cups halved cherry or grape tomatoes

1 large head romaine lettuce, chopped

2 avocados, pitted, peeled, and chopped

Pepita Parmesan

1. To make the dressing : Combine all of the ingredients in a food processor or blender and process until smooth. Set aside.

2. Bring a large pot of water to a boil and cook the pasta according to the package instructions until al dente. Drain, rinse the pasta with cold water, then drain again. Transfer the pasta to a large bowl.

3. Heat a large frying pan, preferably cast iron, over medium heat. Add the chickpeas and liquid aminos and cook, stirring occasionally, until all of the liquid has been absorbed, 4 to 5 minutes. Remove from the heat and add to the pasta.

4. Let the chickpeas cool for 5 to 10 minutes. Add the tomatoes, lettuce, and dressing and toss until combined. Gently fold in the avocado. Cover and refrigerate for 1 hour, or up to 3 hours, before serving. Serve topped with Pepita Parmesan (you can add it to the large bowl if people are serving themselves, or over individual servings if that's how you're serving it). This is best when eaten the day it's prepared but will keep in an airtight container in the fridge for about 1 day.

Sun-Dried Tomato & White Bean Bruschetta

SERVES 10 TO 12

PREP TIME: 10 minutes
ACTIVE TIME: 15 minutes

1 long vegan baguette (or other crusty bread; gluten-free if necessary)

1½ cups cooked cannellini beans (or one 15-ounce can, rinsed and drained)

¾ cups oil-packed sun-dried tomatoes, well drained and diced small

1 garlic clove, crushed

2 tablespoons fresh basil chiffonade

3 tablespoons white wine vinegar

Salt and black pepper to taste

½ cup toasted pine nuts (or other toasted nut or seed), optional

½ cup chopped green onions, optional

1. Preheat the oven to 350°F. Slice the bread into ½-inch slices and arrange them on a baking sheet. Bake for 7 to 10 minutes, until crispy and toasted. Set aside.

2. While the bread is toasting, mix together the beans, tomatoes, garlic, basil, vinegar, salt, and pepper.

3. Scoop some bean mixture onto each of the toasts and sprinkle the tops with pine nuts and green onions (if using). Serve immediately.

TIP

- You can prepare the bruschetta topping a few hours in advance and chill until ready to use.
- If you have leftover bean mixture, it makes a great filling for a wrap or sandwich.

Chickpea Croquettes with Dill Yogurt Sauce

SERVES 6 TO 8

PREP TIME: 20 minutes
ACTIVE TIME: 50 minutes

dill yogurt sauce

1 cup plain coconut yogurt (or soy yogurt; preferably unsweetened)

6 tablespoons vegan mayonnaise (soy-free if necessary)

¼ cup lemon juice

2 tablespoons freshly chopped dill (or 1 tbsp. dried dill)

2 teaspoons maple syrup (exclude if using sweetened yogurt)

1½ teaspoons garlic powder

1 teaspoon salt

croquettes

1 pound sweet potatoes or yams, peeled and roughly chopped

One 15-oz can chickpeas, brine reserved, chickpeas rinsed and drained

1 tablespoon reserved chickpea brine

4 green onions, finely chopped (green and white parts)

⅔ cup cornmeal (certified gluten-free if necessary)

1 garlic clove, crushed

1 teaspoon grated lemon zest

½ teaspoon paprika

Pinch of cayenne pepper

Salt and black pepper to taste

1 cup vegan panko bread crumbs (gluten-free if necessary)

Olive oil for frying

1. To make the sauce : Stir together the sauce ingredients in a medium bowl. Cover and refrigerate until ready to use.

2. To make the croquettes : Place the sweet potatoes in a pot and cover with water. Bring to a boil and cook for about 7 minutes, until tender. Drain well.

3. Place the chickpeas and 1 tablespoon brine in a large bowl and mash until broken into small pieces. Add the sweet potatoes and mash until mostly smooth. Add the green onions, cornmeal, garlic, lemon zest, paprika, cayenne pepper, salt, and pepper. Stir until combined.

4. Line a baking sheet with parchment paper or a silicone baking mat. Pour the bread crumbs into a shallow bowl. Scoop up an amount of the croquette mixture slightly larger than a golf ball, shape it into a patty, coat it in bread crumbs, and place it on the prepared baking sheet. Repeat with the remaining croquette mixture.

5. Line a plate with paper towels. Heat a large frying pan, preferably cast iron, over medium heat. Add enough olive oil to coat the bottom of the pan and let it heat until it shimmers. Add half of the croquettes and cook for 3 to 4 minutes on each side, until golden. Transfer to the plate to drain. Add more oil to the pan if needed (allow the oil to heat if you add more). Cook the remaining croquettes. Serve warm with the dill yogurt sauce. Leftovers will keep in airtight containers in the fridge for 2 to 3 days.

Champagne Cupcakes

MAKES 12 CUPCAKES

PREP TIME: 10 minutes
ACTIVE TIME: 45 minutes INACTIVE TIME: 40 minutes

cupcakes

2 tablespoons nondairy milk (nut-free and/or soy-free if necessary)

1 tablespoon apple cider vinegar

1¾ cups unbleached all-purpose flour (or gluten-free flour blend, soy-free if necessary)

2 tablespoons arrowroot powder

1 cup coconut sugar

1 teaspoon baking powder

1 teaspoon baking soda

½ teaspoon salt

¼ teaspoon xanthan gum (exclude if using all-purpose flour or if your gluten-free blend includes it)

8 tablespoons vegan butter (soy-free if necessary), at room temperature

⅔ cup vegan Champagne

(or sparkling wine)

1 teaspoon vanilla extract

frosting

8 tablespoons vegan butter (soy-free if necessary)

3 cups powdered sugar (or xylitol)

2 tablespoons vegan Champagne (or sparkling wine)

½ teaspoon cream of tartar

½ teaspoon vanilla extract

Additional vegan decorations, optional

1. **To make the cupcakes** : Preheat the oven to 350°F. Line a 12-cup muffin tin with paper or silicone liners.
2. In a cup or small bowl, stir together the milk and vinegar. Set aside.
3. In a large bowl, whisk together the flour, arrowroot powder, coconut sugar, baking powder, baking soda, salt, and xanthan gum (if using).
4. In a medium bowl, use a hand mixer to cream together the butter and Champagne. Add the milk mixture and vanilla and mix until combined. Slowly add the wet ingredients to the dry ingredients and use the hand mixer to mix until combined.
5. Divide the mixture among the muffin cups and bake for 20 minutes, or until a toothpick inserted into the center comes out clean. Let the cupcakes cool in the muffin tin for 10 minutes before transferring them to a cooling rack to cool completely.
6. While the cupcakes are cooling, **make the frosting** : Use a hand mixer to mix all the frosting ingredients. Refrigerate for at least 15 minutes, or until ready to use.
7. Once the cupcakes are cool, transfer the frosting to a pastry bag fitted with a decorating tip or a large resealable plastic bag with the corner cut out, and use it to pipe frosting onto each cupcake. Alternatively, just use a butter knife or silicone spatula to spread frosting on each cupcake. You can add decorations if you like. Serve immediately or refrigerate until ready to serve. These cupcakes are best the day they're made but will keep in an airtight container in the fridge for 1 to 2 days.

VARIATION

- To make these alcohol-free, replace the Champagne with a vegan ginger ale or sparkling apple cider.

VEGAN BARBEQUES

VEGAN RECIPES BIG ENOUGH TO FEED A CROWD

IN THIS CHAPTER

Deviled Potato Salad

SERVES 4 TO 6

PREP TIME: 10 minutes
ACTIVE TIME: 15 minutes
INACTIVE TIME: 60 minutes

1 pound baby Yukon gold potatoes (or baby Dutch Yellow Potatoes), quartered

¼ cup vegan mayonnaise (soy-free if necessary)

2 tablespoons vegan sweet pickle relish

1 tablespoon yellow mustard (gluten-free if necessary)

2 teaspoons apple cider vinegar

½ teaspoon onion powder

½ teaspoon garlic powder

½ teaspoon paprika, plus more for dusting

½ teaspoon black salt (kala namak; or regular salt)

1. Place the potatoes in a pot and cover with water. Bring to a boil and cook the potatoes until easily pierced with a fork, 7 to 8 minutes. Drain, then rinse the potatoes with cold water until cool. Drain well.

2. Combine the mayonnaise, relish, mustard, vinegar, onion powder, garlic powder, paprika, and salt in a large bowl and stir until combined. Fold in the potatoes, letting them get mashed a little along the way. Lightly dust the top of the salad with more paprika and refrigerate for 1 hour before serving. Leftovers will keep in an airtight container in the fridge for 3 to 4 days.

Herbed Tofu Burgers

MAKES 6 BURGERS

PREP TIME: 10 minutes
ACTIVE TIME: 45 minutes
INACTIVE TIME: 30 minutes

1 teaspoon olive oil

1 cup chopped yellow onion

2 garlic cloves, minced

One 14-ounce block extra firm tofu, pressed for about 30 minutes

2 tablespoons liquid aminos (or gluten-free tamari)

1 teaspoon v egan Worcestershire sauce (gluten-free if necessary)

½ teaspoon liquid smoke

½ teaspoon ground cumin

½ teaspoon dried thyme

½ teaspoon dried oregano

½ teaspoon dried basil

½ teaspoon dried parsley

¾ cup rolled oats (certified gluten-free if necessary)

½ cup vegan bread crumbs (gluten-free if necessary)

2 tablespoons sesame seeds

Salt and black pepper to taste

Olive oil spray

6 vegan burger buns (gluten-free if necessary)

Burger fixings (all are optional): lettuce, sliced tomato, sliced avocado, sliced red onion, pickles, Pickled Red Cabbage & Onion Relish , ketchup, mustard, barbecue sauce, Basic Cashew Cheese Sauce or other vegan cheese

1. Heat the olive oil in a large frying pan over medium heat. Add the onion and garlic and sauté until the onion is translucent.

2. Transfer to a food processor. Add the tofu, liquid aminos, Worcestershire sauce, liquid smoke, cumin, thyme, oregano, basil, parsley, and ¼ cup of the oats. Process until smooth.

3. Transfer the mixture to a large bowl and add the remaining oats, the bread crumbs, and sesame seeds. Mix until combined. Add salt and pepper.

4. Line a baking sheet with parchment paper or a silicone baking mat. Divide the mixture into six equal parts. Using your hands or a greased biscuit cutter (sized to fit the buns), form the mixture into patties and place on the baking sheet.

5. Heat a large grill pan or frying pan, preferably cast iron, over medium heat. Generously spray the pan with olive oil. Place 2 or 3 patties in the pan (however many will fit without being crowded) and cook for 4 to 5 minutes on each side, a few minutes longer if your patties are more than ¾ inch thick, until firm, crisp, and browned on the outside. Place the burgers on buns. Repeat with the remaining patties, respraying the pan between batches.

6. Let everyone assemble their burger with their choice of fixings. Leftover burgers will keep in an airtight container in the fridge for up to 4 days.

Ranch-Seasoned Corn on the Cob

SERVES 4, WITH EXTRA SEASONING

PREP TIME: 5 minutes
ACTIVE TIME: 25 minutes INACTIVE TIME: 15 minutes

ranch seasoning

2 tablespoons dried parsley

1 tablespoon dried minced onion

2 teaspoons onion powder

2 teaspoons garlic powder

1½ teaspoons dried dill

1½ teaspoons dried oregano

1 teaspoon celery seed

1 teaspoon salt

1 teaspoon coconut sugar

½ teaspoon paprika

¼ teaspoon black pepper

corn on the cob

At least 4 ears corn, in the husks (1 or more per person)

Vegan butter (soy-free if necessary)

Chopped fresh parsley, optional

1. To make the ranch seasoning : Combine all the ingredients in a food processor or spice grinder. Pulse a couple of times until it's a coarse powder. Transfer to a jar or airtight container.

2. To make the corn on the cob : Peel back the husks of the corn without detaching them. Remove and discard all the silk. Pull the husks back over the corn and place the ears in a large bowl or pot of cold water. Soak for 15 minutes.

3. Heat the grill to medium-high or heat a grill pan on the stove over medium heat. Place the corn on the grill and cook for 20 minutes, flipping once halfway through, or until the husks are slightly charred and the corn is tender.

4. If you want pretty grill marks on the corn, peel back the husks, place the corn directly on the grill, and cook for a couple of minutes on each side. Otherwise, just remove the corn from the grill.

5. Use a kitchen towel to pull back the husks. Tie them to form a handle. Spread butter over each ear and season generously with ranch seasoning. Sprinkle with chopped parsley (if desired) and serve immediately.

VARIATION

You can also roast the corn. Remove the husks when you remove the silk and skip the soaking. Place each ear on a sheet of aluminum foil. Spread butter on the corn, then sprinkle generously with the ranch seasoning. Wrap the aluminum tightly around the corn. Roast at 450°F for 15 to 20 minutes, until the corn is tender.

TIP You will have leftover spice blend, but don't worry—you can use this ranch seasoning just as you would any spice blend! Use it in the marinade for the Grilled Veggie Kebabs , sprinkle on the Perfect Roasted Potatoes before they go in the oven, or top your Quick & Easy Avocado Toast with it.

Creamy, Crunchy Coleslaw

SERVES 10 TO 12

PREP TIME: 15 minutes
ACTIVE TIME: 20 minutes
INACTIVE TIME: 35 minutes

1 medium (1½- to 2-poundhead green cabbage, quartered, cored, and shredded on a mandoline or grater

2 medium carrots, peeled and grated

¾ cup vegan sugar

½ cup kosher salt

3 or 4 green onions, chopped (green and white parts)

¾ cup vegan mayonnaise (soy-free if necessary)

¼ cup apple cider vinegar

2 tablespoons maple syrup

2 teaspoons Dijon mustard (gluten-free if necessary)

1 teaspoon dried parsley

1 teaspoon celery seed

1 teaspoon black pepper

Salt to taste

1. Combine the cabbage and carrots in a large bowl and toss with the sugar and kosher salt. Let rest for 5 minutes, then transfer to a colander and rinse thoroughly with cold water. (Not thoroughly rinsing the cabbage will result in overly salty slaw.) Rinse and dry the bowl. Run the cabbage and carrots through a salad spinner to remove the excess moisture, or spread out the mixture on a clean kitchen towel and pat dry with paper towels or another kitchen towel. Once dry, return the mixture to the bowl and add the green onions.

2. In a small bowl, mix together the mayonnaise, vinegar, maple syrup, mustard, parsley, celery seed, and pepper. Once thoroughly combined, add the dressing to the cabbage mixture and toss until evenly coated. Add salt if needed. Chill for at least 30 minutes before serving. Leftovers will keep in an airtight container in the fridge for 2 to 3 days.

VEGAN HOLIDAYS

VEGAN DISHES THAT WILL START NEW HOLIDAY TRADITIONS

IN THIS CHAPTER

Cheesy Roasted Sweet Potatoes

SERVES 6 TO 8

PREP TIME: 5 minutes
ACTIVE TIME: 5 minutes
INACTIVE TIME: 35 minutes

4 large sweet potatoes or yams (2 pounds), peeled and diced

Olive oil spray

4 to 6 tablespoons nutritional yeast

1 teaspoon garlic powder

1 teaspoon smoked paprika

Salt and black pepper to taste

1. Preheat the oven to 425°F. Line two baking sheets with parchment paper or silicone baking mats.

2. Spread out the sweet potatoes on the sheets and spray with olive oil. Sprinkle the nutritional yeast, garlic powder, paprika, salt, and pepper over them and toss to coat.

3. Bake for 30 to 35 minutes, until easily pierced with a fork, tossing them once halfway through to ensure even cooking. Serve immediately. Refrigerate leftovers in an airtight container for 3 to 4 days.

Green Bean Casserole with Crispy Onion Topping

SERVES 6 TO 8

PREP TIME: 15 minutes (not including time to make Cream of Mushroom Soup)
ACTIVE TIME: 25 minutes
INACTIVE TIME: 25 minutes

Olive oil spray

1 pound fresh green beans, trimmed

Cream of Mushroom Soup

1 tablespoon vegan butter (soy-free if necessary)

1 sweet onion, quartered and thinly sliced

¾ cup vegan panko bread crumbs (gluten-free if necessary)

½ teaspoon garlic powder

½ teaspoon salt

3 tablespoons nutritional yeast, optional

1. Preheat the oven to 400°F . Lightly spray a 9 × 13-inch baking dish with olive oil.

2. Place the green beans in a steamer basket over a pot of boiling water and cover. Steam for 5 minutes, then transfer to a large bowl. Pour the soup into the bowl and stir to combine. Set aside.

3. While the green beans are steaming, melt half of the butter in a large frying pan over medium heat. Add the onion and cook, stirring occasionally, until soft and golden, 5 to 7 minutes. Transfer the onions to a medium bowl. (Don't bother to clean the pan.) Melt the remaining butter in the frying pan and add the bread crumbs. Cook, stirring frequently, until the crumbs are crispy. Stir in the garlic powder and salt and remove from the heat. Add to the onions along with the nutritional yeast (if using). Stir to combine.

4. Pour the green bean mixture into the prepared baking dish. Spread the onion mixture over the top. Bake for 25 minutes, or until the topping is crispy and the casserole is bubbly. Serve immediately. Leftovers will keep in an airtight container in the fridge for 3 to 4 days.

TIP

To prepare this in advance, bake the casserole without the topping for 25 minutes. Refrigerate until ready to serve. Prepare the onion topping, spread it on the top, and bake the casserole at 400°F for 15 to 20 minutes, until heated through.

Mashed Potatoes

SERVES 8 TO 10

PREP TIME: 10 minutes
ACTIVE TIME: 10 minutes

3 pounds Yukon gold potatoes, peeled and chopped into large chunks

½ cup unsweetened nondairy milk (nut-free and/or soy-free if necessary), plus more if needed

¼ cup olive oil

Salt and black pepper to taste

1. Place the potatoes in a pot and cover with water. Bring to a boil and cook until the potatoes are tender, 7 to 8 minutes. Drain the potatoes, then return them to the pot.

2. Add the milk and olive oil. Mash until it reaches the desired consistency. If the potatoes are still too dry, add milk by the tablespoon until it reaches the desired moisture level. Add salt and pepper. Leftovers will keep in the fridge in an airtight container for up to 4 days.

VARIATIONS

- Truffled Mashed Potatoes: Replace 3 tablespoons of the olive oil with truffle oil, and add ½ teaspoon of garlic powder.

- Reduced-Calorie Mashed Potatoes: Replace half of the potatoes with 1½ pounds cauliflower florets.

TIP

- To make the mashed potatoes extra smooth, process them in a food processor with the milk and olive oil.

Maple-Miso Tempeh Cutlets

SERVES 4

PREP TIME: 5 minutes
ACTIVE TIME: 20 minutes
INACTIVE TIME: 20 minutes

Two 8-ounce packages tempeh

¼ cup low-sodium vegetable broth

¼ cup liquid aminos (or gluten-free tamari)

¼ cup maple syrup

2 teaspoons white soy miso (or chickpea miso)

1 teaspoon dried sage

1 teaspoon dried thyme

Salt and black pepper to taste

1. Chop each tempeh block in half horizontally, then chop each half diagonally so you have eight triangles.

2. Fill a large shallow saucepan with a couple of inches of water and fit with a steamer basket. Place the tempeh triangles in the steamer basket and cover with a lid. Bring to a boil, then reduce to a simmer. Steam the tempeh for 15 to 20 minutes, flipping the triangles once halfway through. Remove the steamer basket from the pan (keep the tempeh in the basket) and set aside.

3. Dump the water from the saucepan. Combine the vegetable broth, liquid aminos, maple syrup, miso, sage, and thyme in the pan and stir to mix. Add the tempeh triangles and bring to a boil. Once boiling, reduce the heat to a low simmer. Let the tempeh simmer in the sauce for 10 to 12 minutes, flipping them once halfway through, until the sauce is absorbed and starts to caramelize. Remove from the heat and add salt and pepper. Serve immediately. Leftovers will keep in an airtight container in the fridge for 4 to 5 days.

TIP

For a killer Thanksgiving Leftovers Sandwich, slice one of the triangles widthwise so that you have two thinner triangles. Use those in the sandwich, along with some Easy Tahini Gravy, Cheesy Roasted Sweet Potatoes, and maybe some Green Bean Casserole with Crispy Onion Topping.

Easy Tahini Gravy

MAKES 3 CUPS

PREP TIME: 5 minutes
ACTIVE TIME: 15 minutes

1 tablespoon vegan butter (soy-free if necessary)

½ yellow onion, finely diced

1 teaspoon minced garlic

½ teaspoon dried thyme

½ teaspoon dried rosemary

2 tablespoons oat flour (certified gluten-free if necessary)

2½ cups low-sodium vegetable broth

2 tablespoons tahini (gluten-free if necessary)

2 tablespoons liquid aminos (or gluten-free tamari; use coconut aminos to be soy-free)

1 tablespoon nutritional yeast

Salt and black pepper to taste

1. Melt the butter in a large shallow saucepan over medium heat. Add the onion and garlic and sauté until the onion is translucent, about 5 minutes. Add the thyme and rosemary and cook for a minute more. Add the flour and cook, stirring continuously, until the flour is completely incorporated.

2. Add the broth, tahini, and liquid aminos and stir until well combined. Cook, stirring frequently, until the gravy is thick and glossy, 5 to 7 minutes. Add the nutritional yeast and remove from the heat.

3. Use an immersion blender to blend the gravy until smooth. You can also transfer the gravy to a blender to blend until smooth. Add salt and pepper. Serve immediately. Leftovers will keep in an airtight container in the fridge for 2 to 3 days.

METRIC CONVERSIONS

The recipes in this book have not been tested with metric measurements, so some variations might occur.

Remember that the weight of dry ingredients varies according to the volume or density factor: 1 cup of flour weighs far less than 1 cup of sugar, and 1 tablespoon doesn't necessarily hold 3 teaspoons.

General Formula for Metric Conversion

Ounces to grams	multiply ounces by 28.35
Grams to ounces	multiply ounces by 0.035
Pounds to grams	multiply pounds by 453.5
Pounds to kilograms	multiply pounds by 0.45
Cups to liters	multiply cups by 0.24
Fahrenheit to Celsius	subtract 32 from Fahrenheit temperature, multiply by 5, divide by 9
Celsius to Fahrenheit	multiply Celsius temperature by 9, divide by 5, add 32

Volume (Liquid) Measurements

1 teaspoon = ⅙ fluid ounce = 5 milliliters

1 tablespoon = ½ fluid ounce = 15 milliliters 2 tablespoons = 1 fluid ounce = 30 milliliters

¼ cup = 2 fluid ounces = 60 milliliters

⅓ cup = 2⅔ fluid ounces = 79 milliliters

½ cup = 4 fluid ounces = 118 milliliters

1 cup or ½ pint = 8 fluid ounces = 250 milliliters

2 cups or 1 pint = 16 fluid ounces = 500 milliliters

4 cups or 1 quart = 32 fluid ounces = 1,000 milliliters

1 gallon = 4 liters

Oven Temperature Equivalents, Fahrenheit (F) and Celsius (C)

100°F = 38°C

200°F = 95°C

250°F = 120°C

300°F = 150°C

350°F = 180°C

400°F = 205°C

450°F = 230°C

Volume (Dry) Measurements

¼ teaspoon = 1 milliliter

½ teaspoon = 2 milliliters

¾ teaspoon = 4 milliliters 1 teaspoon = 5 milliliters

1 tablespoon = 15 milliliters

¼ cup = 59 milliliters

⅓ cup = 79 milliliters

½ cup = 118 milliliters

⅔ cup = 158 milliliters

¾ cup = 177 milliliters 1 cup = 225 milliliters

4 cups or 1 quart = 1 liter

½ gallon = 2 liters 1 gallon = 4 liters

Linear Measurements

½ in = 1½ cm

1 inch = 2½ cm

6 inches = 15 cm

8 inches = 20 cm

10 inches = 25 cm

12 inches = 30 cm

20 inches = 50 cm

CPSIA information can be obtained
at www.ICGtesting.com
Printed in the USA
BVHW091057030521
606332BV00004B/477

9 781802 680614